Colloidal Silver Today

The All-Natural
Wide-Spectrum
Germ Killer

Warren Jefferson

Healthy Living Publications
Summertown, Tennessee

© 2003 Warren Jefferson

Published in the United States by

Healthy Living Publications, an imprint of Book Publishing Company
P.O. Box 99, Summertown, TN 38483
1-888-260-8458

Printed in the United States

14 13 12   11 10   09   9 8 7 6 5

ISBN13   978-1-57067-154-8

Library of Congress Cataloging-in-Publication Data
Jefferson, Warren, 1943-
  Colloidal silver today : the all-natural, wide-spectrum   germ killer
/ by Warren Jefferson.
      p. cm.
Includes bibliographical references.
ISBN 1-57067-154-0
1. Colloidal silver--Therapeutic use--Popular works. 2. Colloidal
silver--Popular works. I. Title.
RM666.S5J44 2003
615'.2654--dc22   2003018238

Book Publishing Co. is a member of Green Press Initiative. We chose to print
this title on paper with postconsumer recycled content, processed without
chlorine, which saved the following natural resources:

BOOK
PUBLISHING
COMPANY

3 trees
74 pounds of solid waste
1,212 gallons of water
252 pounds of greenhouse gases
1 million BTU of net energy

green
press
INITIATIVE

For more information, visit <www.greenpressinitiative.org>. Savings calculations
thanks to the Environmental Defense Paper Calculator, <www.papercalculator.org>.

TABLE OF CONTENTS

Colloidal Silver Today

There is a lot of interest in the germ fighter colloidal silver (CS). If you do a Google search for collloidal silver on the Internet you will be given over 64,000 Web pages to explore. Throughout the world natural health practitioners are using it as an alternative to antibiotic, antiviral, and antifungal products. With it they are treating a host of illnesses and diseases, from minor skin infections to Lyme disease. Individuals too are prescribing CS for themselves and their loved ones, including pets. People use it to treat sick farm animals and horses. CS is becoming the peoples' germicide—cheap, easily manufactured, and effective. In vitro tests conducted in 1999 by a prominent university show that CS kills a broad range of disease microbes including *E. coli, Staphylococcus aureus, Streptococcus pneumonia, Salmonella arizona,* and Anthrax.

When I first heard about CS it really caught my attention. What? Could something so simple and harmless actually destroy that many different germs? I had to know more. So began my quest to learn everything I could about this amazing substance.

The traditional medical establishment knows very little about CS. Most doctors who have heard of it think it's a "risk-with-no-benefit" product and caution against its use. It's politically incorrect to be associated with CS, but this hasn't always been the case.

Almost one hundred years ago, before the discovery of sulfa drugs and antibiotics, CS was considered a high-tech

4

germ fighter and most doctors' offices had CS in their medicine cabinet. They used it to treat many serious medical conditions, including gonorrhea, tonsillitis, whooping cough, typhoid, and others. (Searle 1919)

A few years ago the Food and Drug Administration (FDA) made a ruling regarding CS, stating that it does not recognize CS as being useful in the treatment of any disease. The FDA ruling makes it illegal for manufacturers of CS to claim that their product can cure anything. CS can only be sold as a dietary supplement, which requires less regulation. Although there has been no published, modern scientific testing using double blind studies, the anecdotal evidence that CS cures disease is impressive. People throughout the world use it and swear to its healing ability.

Many people today have lost trust in Western allopathic medicine with its profit motive and the rising cost of prescription drugs. They also are concerned about the overuse of antibiotics and the alarming growth of resistant strains of bacteria that are developing as a result. CS seems to answer these concerns for those who are using it.

Another reason for the appeal of CS is that here is a powerful germ killer not controlled by a pharmaceutical company. No drug company has become interested in CS because there is no financial incentive. It would be difficult to patent a natural element. CS is just silver and water and a very simple process to combine them. There you have it—no high-tech manufacturing process involved. People are attracted to the simplicity of it. You can make it at home!

Throughout this book I will be referring to the type of colloidal silver (CS) created through electrolysis by the low-voltage, direct current method (LVDC). It is composed of pure water, colloidal sized particles of silver, and dissolved silver ions.

CS is sold in most natural food stores across the country and CS generators are available that will enable you to make a good quality product. If you really want to save money, instructions are available on the Internet to make your own CS generator.

In this book you will learn about silver and its early uses dating back thousands of years; the uses of colloidal silver as a germ fighter before antibiotics were developed; the modern medical uses of silver as well as the non-medical uses; the low toxicity of silver and the maximum safe dose; and the current status of CS with the FDA.

You will learn what a colloid is; what CS is and the different products that have been called colloidal silver over the years; how CS is produced; how to identify the best type of CS; and how to make a simple CS generator that will allow you to make CS at home.

You will read testimonials by people who believe they have overcome disease with the help of CS. There also is a discussion of the problem of drug-resistant bacteria. Finally you will be given a list of resources where you can buy CS and find more information about it.

I do not have a financial interest in CS or promote the use of it. I took an interest in CS after reading about its use long ago to fight germs and infection and about people using it today to successfully treat serious illness. If what people say about CS is true, it could be a powerful new (rediscovered) tool to help humankind fight deadly microbes. Considering all the positive reports from people using CS, it seems that the time has come for it to be thoroughly researched and information made available to the general public.

With this book I have attempted to compile as much information as possible from reliable and primary sources about the usage, effectiveness, and safety of silver and CS. I hope this information will help anyone who is considering using CS make an informed decision.

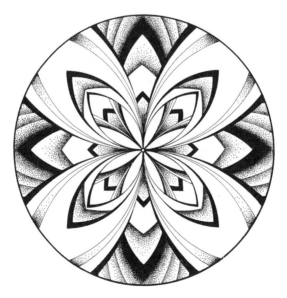

SILVER THE METAL

CS is a fascinating substance. It is basically silver and water. But ingredients combined often are more than the sum of their parts. First there is silver, a precious metal, and water, the universal solvent, in a colloidal state. What is a colloidal state? To answer this question let's turn to science, and start with some basic facts about silver.

Silver is a naturally occurring, comparatively rare metal found in the earth's crust. It is the sixty-seventh most abundant natural element. It is soft, white, malleable, and ductile (can be drawn into wire). Discovered in ancient times (there is no known date of discovery for silver) it is mentioned in Genesis, and the Greeks smelted it out of lead early in their history. It's the forty-seventh element in the periodic chart (which means it has forty-seven electrons) with the symbol Ag and atomic weight 108. It has the highest thermal and electrical conductivity of all metals with the lowest contact resistance. It is not soluble in water and does not combine easily with other elements to form compounds, hence the "noble" metal designation. Silver tarnishes but the structure of the metal is not weakened as with iron. Silver is often found as a by-product during the mining of copper, lead, zinc, and gold, primarily in the United States, Peru, and Mexico. As a precious metal, its value has fluctuated over the years, reaching a high in the 1980s.

EARLY USES OF SILVER

It has been known for centuries that silver has powerful germ killing properties. In ancient civilizations, the wealthy used silver containers to store liquids, and silver eating utensils were the most preferred. There are reports from long ago of silver rods being applied into open wounds to stave off infection.

[In traditional Ayurvedic medicine, a healing system that originated in India over 2000 years ago], silver is used in ash form and in its suspended form, colloidal, to rejuvenate the body. It helps with liver and infectious conditions, as well as inflammatory conditions. (www.ayurveda.com)

CS was developed circa 1891 and was used to treat scores of infectious ailments. It was taken orally and used as a throat gargle, injected intravenously and intramuscularly, used as eye drops, and applied topically.

Albert Searle, the founder of the pharmaceutical company that later became Merck, was a researcher and proponent of CS in the early 1900s. In his book *The Use of Colloids in Health and Disease*, he presents his findings on the curative effects of CS and reviews numerous articles published in the *British Medical Journal* and *Lancet* on the successful use of CS in curing disease. Searle writes, "The germicidal action of certain metals in the colloidal state having been demonstrated, it only remained to apply them to the human subject, and this has been done in a large number of cases with astonishingly successful results. . . for internal administration, either orally or hypodermically, they have the advantage of being rapidly fatal to the parasites—both bacterial and otherwise—without any toxic action on the host." (page 75)

Colloidal Silver Today

From Macleod we learn about the successful treatments for follicular tonsillitis, conjunctivitis, gonorrheal conjunctivitis, impetigo, septic ulcers of the legs, ringworm of body, soft sores, pustular eczema of the scalp, boils, gonorrhea, and other conditions. (Searle, page 83)

"Sir James Cantlie found it [CS] particularly effective in cases of sprue, dysentery, and intestinal troubles. Sir Malcolm Morris has found that CS is free from the drawbacks of other preparations of silver, indeed, instead of producing irritation it has a distinctly soothing effect. It rapidly subdues inflammation and promotes the healing of the lesions." He goes on to write, "Collosol argentum (CS) has been used successfully for curing influenza as well as preventing it when sprayed into the nostrils, bathing the eyes, and as a gargle for the throat." (Searle, page 83)

Silver compounds have been employed for medical uses for centuries. In the nineteenth and early twentieth centuries, silver arsphenamine was used in the treatment of syphilis. (U.S. EPA IRIS 1996)

In 1914, Henry Crookes experimented with CS and reported "metals (in what is now called the colloidal state) kill the bacteria only, and exercise a bland and soothing effect on the animal tissues." In laboratory experiments in vitro he used "collosol" silver, as he called it, in a concentration of one part in 2000 and found that *B. tuberculosis* was killed in four minutes and *Streptococci* and other pathogenic organisms were killed in three or four minutes. "I know of no microbe that is not killed in laboratory experiments in six minutes." He was convinced

10

that CS should be investigated thoroughly and given extended trials by the medical profession.

It is to be hoped that they [colloidal metals] will receive the attention which they deserve. (Crookes 1914)

Silver preparations during this early time were produced by a number of manufacturers and were called by various product names: Argenti Acetas, Albargin, Argonin, Argyn, Argyrol, Largin, Lunosol, Novargan, Proganol, and Silvol, among others.

Three types of products containing silver were used by doctors during this time—mild silver protein and silver salts both of which are irritating to animal tissue, and electro colloidal silver water. Mild silver protein and silver salt preparations have a silver concentration of 10 percent and higher. This high concentration of silver in some cases led to a condition called *argyria*, a permanent but benign blue-gray coloring of the skin. The high concentration of silver in these early products makes comparisons with modern day CS useless.

In 1938 with the development of cheaper sulfa drugs and later when penicillin became widely available, CS fell out of favor. By 1970 the major pharmaceutical companies no longer produced CS and it was no longer listed in any medical treatment reference book.

Colloidal Silver Today

CLINICAL USES OF SILVER

The most common use of silver preparations today is as germ fighting agents in the treatment of serious burn wounds in both humans and animals. A related use is as a coating for nylon fabric to cover burn wounds and traumatic injuries. A silver delivery dressing called Acitcoat®, a three-ply gauze wound dressing that releases silver for at least forty-eight hours, is recommended by Burnsurgery.org, an organization committed to educating burn care professionals around the world. Another company, Argentum Medical, manufactures wound dressings that employ a silver-plated fabric called Silverlon®. Silverlon®-based products are antibacterial, antifungal, and hypoallergenic.

There are reports of silver ions having a stimulating effect on tissue regeneration in serious wounds using silver plated fabric and low voltage electricity. Two silver electrodes are used. One is placed in contact with the wound and the other on adjacent intact tissue. A small DC electrical current is passed between them releasing ions into the wound. This causes ordinary cells to change into specialized cells for bone and tissue regeneration. (Becker et al. 1998) (See Appendix C.)

A diluted solution of silver nitrate is used as drops in the eyes of newborn babies to prevent neonatal eye infections. Blood-contacting catheters coated with silver have been used with great success and are ten times more effective in retarding infections compared to non-silver catheters, with little or no problems with biocompatibility. (Silver Institute, Bakteriol, 1995)

It is somewhat of a mystery as to how silver kills a microorganism. Crookes speculated that a microbe, which is many hundreds of times larger than a CS particle and has a charge opposite it, would attract many thousands of CS particles, and this would likely be the cause of its death.

Silver ion is a very toxic substance when viewed from the standpoint of its action as an inhibitor of enzymes and as a metabolic inhibitor of lower forms of life. Biochemically, silver ions (Ag+) can act as a potent enzyme inhibitor. (Chambers et al. 1974)

NONCLINICAL USES OF SILVER

Silver is used throughout the world to purify water. Hospitals and hotels use silver filters in their water distribution systems to control infectious agents. Silver filters are used to sterilize recycled water aboard the MIR space station and the NASA space shuttle. Silver is used to purify swimming pool water. A line of home- water purification units sold in the U.S. uses silverized activated carbon filters, and Potters for Peace use silver in a low-tech third world water filter. It is used in lozenges and chewing gum to help people stop smoking. In Mexico a silver product is used to disinfect vegetables and drinking water. In the United Kingdom a slow-release silver compound is used as a preservative in some brands of cosmetics and toiletries. In Japan, a silver compound is mixed into plastics for antimicrobial protection of telephone receivers, calculators, toilet seats, and children's toys. Metallic silver-copper ceramic disks are sold as an alternative to laundry detergents. (Association for the Prudent Use of Antibiotics newsletter, 1999)

Tests done at the University of Florida's Institute of Food and Agricultural Sciences demonstrate the effectiveness of silver and copper ions in killing harmful bacteria in oyster tanks. Oysters quite frequently develop bacteria problems, causing the loss of valuable product. Here is an efficient and ecological way to solve this problem without harming the oysters. Silver ionization also is being used by chicken farmers to reduce bacteria and fungus problems in their flocks. (The Silver Institute)

DRUG-RESISTANT MICROBES

A report issued by the National Institute of Allergies and Infectious Diseases states the following:

> Drug-resistant infectious agents—those that are not killed or inhibited by antimicrobial compounds—are an increasingly important public health concern. Tuberculosis, gonorrhea, malaria, and childhood ear infections are just a few of the diseases that have become more difficult to treat due to the emergence of drug-resistant pathogens. Antimicrobial resistance is becoming a factor in virtually all hospital-acquired infections. Many physicians are concerned that several bacterial infections soon may be untreatable. (NIAID)

The report goes on to say that the costs for treating antibiotic-resistant infections in the United States may be as high as $30 billion. Resistant strains of *Staphylococcus aureus* are a big problem in hospitals across this country. There are only a few drugs that are effective against this microorganism, one of which is vancomycin. Yet there are recent reports of vancomycin-resistant *S. aureus* strains in Japan and the United States.

Streptococcus pneumoniae, the disease microbe that causes thousands of cases of meningitis and pneumonia, and millions of cases of ear infections in the United States each year, is developing a resistance to penicillin, the drug of choice by most doctors. Unfortunately, many of these penicillin-resistant strains also are resistant to other antibiotics. (NIAID)

Multidrug-resistant strains of tuberculosis (MDR-TB) have been evolving over the last ten years. This is a serious threat to people infected with HIV. Three million people a year die from diarrheal diseases in third world countries. Resistant strains of bacteria, such as *Shigella dysenteriae, Campylobacter, Vibrio cholerae, Escherichia coli,* and *Salmonella* are emerging, causing increased suffering. (NIAID)

The rising use of antifungal drugs has caused concern that fungi will develop a drug resistance. In fact there has been a recent report of a species that is resistant to fluconazole, a popular drug used to treat candidia, a systemic fungal disease. (NIAID)

Scientists are no longer able to develop new antibiotics as quickly as before. We could be in for an extremely difficult period in our fight against deadly disease microbes as they build resistances to the current line of antibiotics.

Resistance to Silver

The oft-stated claim by some manufacturers and proponents of CS that microbes cannot develop a resistance to CS may not be true. A case of silver resistance was reported by the burn ward at Massachusetts General Hospital. Three patients there died from an Ag+ resistant *Salmonella* strain. (Gupta et al., cited by APUA newsletter, 1999)

Consider this: thriving bacteria colonies have been found in silver mines. This bacteria was collected and isolated by a scientific team from Sweden. They grew the bacteria together with high concentrations of silver, in the form of silver nitrate, and studied the resulting cells using an electron microscope. They discovered that this bacteria is able to store silver in an outer wall of its cell structure and thus be isolated from the usual toxic effects.

The wide and rather uncontrolled use of silver products may result in increased resistance, analogous to the emergence of antibiotic and other biocide-resistant bacteria. Undermining the benefits of these compounds would be unfortunate to the clinical and hygienic uses that depend on the microcidal properties of silver. (Gupta et al., cited by APUA Newsletter, 1999)

NIAID supports research into new and emerging infectious diseases, how a microorganism develops drug resistance, as well as new or improved therapeutics for disease treatment and prevention. In 1998 they had a research budget of $13 million. Part of their mandate is to encourage basic research to identify new classes of antimicrobial agents and develop alternative treatments for drug-resistant infections.

Perhaps with all the money committed to research by the NIAID in their fight against germs, a portion could be spent in research on CS. Its ability to kill infectious agents, toxicity, and silver resistance should be thoroughly examined. CS is not the final answer but it could help.

COLLOIDS

The term *colloid* was first used by the father of colloid chemistry, Thomas Graham (1805-1869), to refer to tiny particles suspended in a liquid or gel that would not pass through a parchment membrane. Those that did pass through such as salt, sugar, and other crystalline substances he called *crystalloids*. The word colloid is derived from the Greek word *kolla* meaning glue. This early definition is too restrictive, and today a colloid is determined more by the size of its particles than by anything else. (Schramm 2001)

Webster's Third New International Dictionary defines a colloid as "any substance (as an aggregate of atoms or molecules), whether a gas, liquid, or solid, in a fine state of subdivision with particles too small to be visible in an ordinary optical microscope that is dispersed in a gas, liquid, or solid medium and does not settle or settles very slowly (as the liquid droplets of fog, solid particles in smoke, bubbles in foam, or gold particles in ruby glass). "

Colloidal particles range from 1 micron to .001 micron in size. One micron equals 1000 nanometer (nm) or one billionth of a meter. (The thickness of a human hair is 76,200 nanometers.) They are larger than molecules but too small to be seen with a microscope. Colloidal particles will scatter a beam of light as, for example when a car headlight can be seen shining through fog at night. This is called the "Tyndall effect." However, the particles do not affect the freezing point, boiling point, or vapor tension of the medium in which they are suspended. (See Appendix A for more information.)

17

COLLOIDAL SILVER

While a colloid can have many forms, colloidal silver is one type of colloid that consists of solid particles suspended in a liquid. The solid is very small particles of metallic silver and the liquid is water. Very small particles in this context refer to particles whose diameter is measured in nanometers. A silver colloid then must have silver particles in suspension. Colloidal silver also contains another form of silver called ions. (Gibbs 1990)

The difference between solutions, colloids, and suspensions is defined by the size of the particles:

solutions $< 10^{-9}$ m (less than 1 nm)
colloids $= 10^{-9}$ m to 10^{-6} m (1 nm to 1000 nm)
suspensions $> 10^{-6}$ m (greater than 1000 nm) (Key 2000)

Different Types of CS

In the past, the term CS was used to describe at least three different substances that contained silver: mild silver protein, silver salts, and electro colloidal silver water. The concentration of silver varies widely in these different products, as does the ratio of particles to silver ions. The effect on the body and the toxicity varies as well. When we come across information about CS, it is important to understand what type of CS is being discussed, especially when the information is negative.

The term CS does not really have a scientific meaning today. It has become a generic term that refers to health products containing silver particles, silver ions, and water. Our discussion will focus on this type of colloidal silver (CS) and its effects in treating disease and infection. I will identify and describe briefly the other types because they are discussed in

18

the medical literature and are still used today. The negative effects that we hear about CS are the result of using the silver salts and mild silver proteins, not electro colloidal silver.

Electro Colloidal Silver (CS)—produced by low-voltage electrolysis in distilled water and the electro-arc process called the Bredig method with deionized water. Both methods produce CS consisting of microscopic (colloidal size) particles of silver suspended in pure water along with dissolved silver ions. Its appearance is transparent clear or transparent with a slight yellow tint, depending on the particle size.

Mild Silver Protein (MSP)—micro particles of silver chemically bound to a protein molecule. Typically made by mixing silver nitrate, sodium hydroxide, and gelatin. It comes in a concentration of 19 to 23 percent silver. The protein molecule acts as a stabilizer to keep the silver particles from combining with each other and settling out. (Gibbs 1990)

Silver Salts (SS)—produced chemically or electrochemically, such as silver nitrate, silver phosphate, silver iodine, and silver chloride. Silver salts tend to be irritating to tissue. Concentrations are between 100 to 500 parts per million (ppm). *MSP* and *SS* are silver compounds, not colloids.

The Ideal Colloidal Silver

There is disagreement among researchers and manufacturers about whether CS's healing ability is caused chiefly by silver particles, silver ions, or both. Consequently there is disagreement as to what CS should be called. (For a kill test comparing various CS products go to: www. natural-immunogenics.com.)

Some think "ionic silver water" is a more accurate term, since in a typical CS product more than 75 percent of the silver is ionic and dissolved. Others think it should be called "electrically isolate silver" or "isolated silver" for the same reason. It may be a misnomer, but the term colloidal silver (CS) persists and is generally used by people in the industry to refer to electrochemically produced colloidal silver containing water, silver particles, and silver ions.

After reviewing the information available, I have concluded that a high quality CS product would have a concentration between 5 and 10 ppm and contain 5 to 10 percent silver particles and correspondingly 90 to 95 percent dissolved ionic silver. It should not contain any other substance. The silver will not necessarily be listed this way on the bottle, however. You may have to ask the manufacturer for product analysis information. The following information is from two contemporary scientists who have researched CS.

> The ideal colloidal silver product [CS] would be made up of particles less than 0.1 micron (um) and preferably ranging from 0.01 to 0.001 um. Since it is desirable to have pure colloidal silver only, the product should be in pure distilled water with no additional dissolved substances. There should be no solids other than silver particles, including no gelatin stabilizers nor other extraneous material, present by accident or design. (Gibbs 1990)

> Colloidal silver contains two forms of silver: metallic silver particles and ions. The total silver is the silver concentration in parts per million and is the measure of ions and silver particles. In a typical product silver ions make up 75 to 99 percent and the particles make up 1 to 25 percent of total silver. A pure silver colloid would be 100 percent silver particles with no ions present. (Key 2000)

Color is another indicator of quality. A yellow product indicates the presence of some additional substance or large particles of silver. High quality CS should be clear and colorless. The pH of CS should be neutral, as close to pH 7 as possible—not an acid or a base. (Gibbs 1990)

When it comes to buying CS, consumers are left to fend for themselves. There are no industry standards of quality for manufacturers producing CS, and there is no government information for consumers. Product quality varies widely among scores of manufacturers. But there are reputable dealers who conduct regular testing on their products and they publish these reports for their customers. If no reports are available, have the product you are considering tested to determine ppm, pH, and conductance. (See Appendix D for a list of testing companies.) When you find a quality product, stick with that manufacturer and pass the word to your friends.

Another way to assure a quality product is to create it yourself. It's not that difficult. You can purchase a generator or make your own generator from the plans in this book. I made my own CS generator and have produced clear, high quality, 10 ppm CS.

The silver-list is a moderated Internet chat group for CS. Much of the discussion centers on how to obtain the best CS. The participants exchange information on techniques, brewing times, and quality, much like the folks who make their own beer or wine. Some people get quite technical and figure ppm using Faraday's electrolysis equation and use columbs verses time curves. Some even calculate the number of ions that come off a square nanometer of silver wire per second. Now this is all beyond me. I just send my CS out to be tested to determine quality.

TESTIMONIALS

Below are testimonials from a number of people using CS. In the spirit of helping others they share their stories of healing. I have made personal contact with each of these people to confirm their stories. None sells CS.

Steven J. Geigle

Prior to using CS I suffered from chronic sinusitis, occasional bronchitis and pneumonia, seasonal allergies, and a little asthma too. I became quite expert at diagnosing my own pneumonia. The docs would swear I didn't have it, but sure enough, after the x-ray, they would have to admit I was right.

In my personal research, I have found that to make CS work, it has to actually interact with the cause of the infection. So for sinusitis I introduce the CS as a mist into the sinus cavities. For respiratory illness I introduce CS into the lungs using a nebulizer. For ear infections CS drops do the job quite well. If I feel any "systemic" symptoms coming on —such as aches, chills, and so forth—I drink a few ounces every half hour for a few hours to increase the level of CS throughout my body. For eye infections, I spray CS directly into the eye, which is not only soothing but quickly reduces the infection. For cuts, I merely place a couple of drops of CS on the pad of a bandage and cover the cut. I don't see any inflammation whatsoever and healing occurs much more quickly. Using these methods, I've been able to effectively prevent various bacterial and/or viral invasions through the years.

Just a few weeks ago my grandson brought home from pre-school a nice full-blown cold. Of course, everyone was exposed. As soon as I felt a scratch in my throat I began taking CS. This time I nebulized and the infection was quickly halted within only two days. I rarely suffer from any illness and never from allergies or asthma anymore.

The FDA says that since I've used CS for a prolonged period I should have a condition called argyria. [see page 32] Frankly, I don't know any CS user that has or is suffering any symptoms whatsoever of argyria from correctly ingesting pure CS. Pure CS is not a silver compound, (such as that used by Rosemary Jacobs who developed argyria) nor a solid (such as silver dust or oxide) and therefore should not be a cause of argyria, but I guess the FDA has yet to see the difference.

It doesn't matter to me what the FDA, the FTC, Quackwatch, or any other group claims. My research and personal use proves to me that colloidal silver works! I encourage you to spend some time surfing my Website for information on colloidal silver. Don't just take my word or the word of others. Test it yourself.

Steven J. Geigle
Portland, Oregon

Warren Jefferson

I once had a Jack Russell Terrier named Jack who loved to chase squirrels.

When I came home from work one evening I noticed he was limping as he came to greet me. I examined him and found a puncture wound on his shoulder. I assumed it was the result of a fight with a squirrel. (I later found a dead one in the yard.) As I picked him up to bring him into the house he yelped in distress. It was obviously a very painful injury. I put him in his bed and he just laid there shivering.

I immediately got the CS and applied it into the wound and gave him about a quarter of an ounce orally. I continued this treatment every half hour for the next three or four hours until I went to bed. He seemed so sick I wasn't sure he would survive the night.

When I got up the next morning, to my pleasant surprise, he greeted me as usual, jumping around at my feet ready to go outside. He was putting his full weight on the injured shoulder. So I opened the door and out he ran into the yard looking for the nearest squirrel to chase. I was amazed how quickly and completely he recovered.

I have a mixed boxer now who sometimes develops weepy eyes. I find that applying a few drops of CS in the affected eye two times a day for a couple of days clears it up nicely.

warren@bookpubco.com

Nancy DeLise

I had relapsing, remitting multiple sclerosis (MS) for thirty-one years. Around 1995 it changed to secondary progressive MS. Thus began my long road of decline. Every day I got worse. When I discovered CS I could barely walk. I was beginning to use a cane. I could not even go up on the curb without aid. My prognosis was grim. I had some knowledge of the great properties of silver, so the idea of CS intrigued me. I researched CS. What did I have to lose?

I began drinking sixteen ounces per day. In about three weeks I began to notice a difference. After the first year I seemed to reach a plateau. I did not improve, but I never got worse.

In August 2001 I had an MRI and it showed I no longer had MS. I have had no new lesions for well over a year. Since the damage is to the myelin and not the central nervous system, I was quite confident I could improve. The following is a diary of my progress:

Eighteen months: I have researched adding hydrogen peroxide to the CS—one drop of 3 percent H_2O_2 per two ounces of CS. I learned this would cause the tiny silver particles to break up into even more minute particles. After fifteen minutes the peroxide is evaporated out of the CS so it is not harmful to the body, but the tinier particles of silver get into the bloodstream quicker. Previously it had been a slow process because by the time the silver got to the myelin where it was needed, it was so diluted it couldn't penetrate the lesions and kill the mycoplasma (MS virus).

Within one week I began to feel the old symptoms again. This is what I call a healing crisis [see Herx reaction, page

46]. I would get symptoms of the MS as the virus was dying and the dying pathogens aggravated the nerves, so for two to four days I would feel as though I was having varying degrees of exacerbation. After a short period, it would end and I was improved again. If I had known about this earlier, I am convinced my recovery time would have decreased a great deal.

One year, nine months: I am sure there is a way for my recovery to go even quicker. I began to research intravenous drips. I worked on this project for about six weeks. I finally found someone with a protocol of infusing CS intravenously. I also found a doctor willing to work with me and give this a try.

One year, eleven months: I had my first IV. By that evening I had my first healing crisis; my legs became extremely heavy (just like they had been two years ago). My fingerstips were still numb, but the numbness was extremely exaggerated. All was better by day four.

Second IV one week later: My legs again are aching a great deal, the numbness in my fingers is very intense. It almost feels like they are not attached to me. All better by day three.

Third, fourth, fifth IV: Each time I experienced a reverse of some symptoms I had either forgotten about over the last forty years or didn't realize were actually MS symptoms. I've practically no problems at all. I feel better then I have in fifteen years. I will have no more IVs, but I will never stop drinking CS. If I had known about the IVs I probably would have had a full recovery even sooner. I am quite sure the old lesions are going away. I am anxious for another MRI to prove this.

Two Year Anniversary: very few symptoms.

I am completely convinced CS will help anyone with an autoimmune disease. I would be happy to share what I've learned with anyone.

Nancy DeLise
380 Blackawk Road
Riverside, Il. 60546
nancymike@prodigy.net

Jason Eaton

I discovered CS out of desperation when a family member was dying in the hospital from a massive flesh-eating bacterial infection (*pseudomona* and *staph* antibiotic-resistant hospital strains) that turned septic. She had a fever of 105 degrees for twenty-one days straight, required blood transfusions during the last week (low levels of oxygen in the blood), and did not respond to even the newest, most aggressive antibiotic treatments (at the time, the "Gorilla Three" failed, and the surgeon elected to utilize Trovan, with equally dismal results). They would take her to surgery every day, sometimes twice daily, to surgically remove infected tissues. I spent at least two weeks writing research institutions and researching allopathic means to address her condition, with no success.

Finally I found CS information through a search on the Internet, and after two days of experimentation, I concluded that the product I was coming up with was acceptable colloidal silver. I snuck it into the hospital in the middle of the night and administered it to her orally, about four to six ounces that first night, and about the same amount twice the next day. Then, between forty-eight and seventy-two hours later, her fever broke for the first time in at least three weeks.

Four days after the fever broke, she came home with a big hole in her stomach about the size of a football that was covered with a temporary skin graft taken from both legs.

Two months later, after healing at a rate that shocked her plastic surgery team (they wanted to wait about eight months to do medical reconstructive surgery), she went back into surgery. From then on it was pretty clear sailing, although the road to health through such an experience can be long and arduous due to the toxicity of the many drugs.

Today I attribute the rapid effect of the colloidal silver to the fact that she had not eaten any solid foods for about one and one-half months and was eating only through intravenous solution; there were no stomach acids present, which was a great advantage.

I'm sold on colloidal silver applications and have been doing my own experiments with external CS formulas for the purpose of tissue regeneration with good success.

While it might be pure coincidence that she recovered just after beginning internal CS treatment, I do not believe this to be the case. Her condition was desperate. Her doctor was one of the state's best specialists, and all he could do was throw his hands up in the air and continue to do the same thing. Was he expecting different results? I'm certain that if it wasn't for the CS she would have died.

Jason R. Eaton
www.silvermedicine.org

Karen Sanders

(nutritionist for humans and animals for over twenty years.)

After using CS for only several weeks, I have some good reports. My husband Sam and I have greatly increased energy, and we've noticed that CS heals scratches and insect bites almost overnight. CS also gives wonderful pain relief when applied topically.

Last Saturday night I got a nasty cat bite on my hand while helping one of the new critters. With blood flowing, I ran for the CS and placed several drops in the puncture wound. After a few minutes, I washed the wound thoroughly with soap and applied more CS. I soaked a cotton pad with CS and taped it over the wound. By Sunday, half of my hand was swollen, inflamed, and sore, but as long as I kept soaking the cotton pad with CS, the pain was relieved. By Sunday night I could move my hand freely and was able to prepare thirty pounds of food for my animals.

I continued to soak the cotton pad covering the wound in the CS. Monday morning the swelling was almost gone and there was no infection. By Tuesday the wound was almost completely closed and there was hardly any inflammation. Normally this type of deep muscle puncture wound would take two to three miserable weeks to heal this well.

Since we received the CS, we've also been giving it to the animals in food and sometimes in their water. I am thrilled to report that two cats with chronic illnesses are no longer taking the destructive steroidal drugs. The kitty with pancreatitis has not vomited once, and her coat is improving every day. The kitty with conjunctivitis has had no symptoms either and is full of energy. I did not use the CS in her eye, just in her food and water. As a nutritionist, I take care to feed the animals a natural, healthy diet, with supplements and enzymes added to their food.

We now are making our own CS and just started giving it to family, friends, and co-workers. After only a few days, one of Sam's co-workers with many allergies and serious fatigue already has more energy and feels noticeably better. She said, "Even my dog has more energy." My sister applied it to a cut, and the cut was nearly healed the next day.

wealthofhealth@webtv.net

Robert Berger
(Unfortunatly Robert passed away in 2007)

I am eighty-one years old and I take an ounce of CS as a prophylactic twice a day, once in the morning and evening. I hold it in my mouth for about five minutes and then swallow it. One of my daughters-in-law had double mastectomy due to cancer and, as the healing process started, one of her nipples turned black. The doctors told her that it was dead tissue and she would lose it. She had seen the pictures of Dr A. B. Flick's work (www.silverlon.com) and had been using CS for some time. After her operation she started her own protocol for healing. She submerged the affected nipple in a small cup of CS for fifteen minutes three times a day. She also kept the bandages moist with CS, throughout the healing process. After three weeks of treatment, the black nipple fell off and there in its place was a brand new, pink nipple. The doctors were amazed at the regeneration.

Nancy Estes

I have a young male rottweiler named Emil who has irritable bowel disease (IBD). This is known to lead to an overgrowth of intestinal bacteria, which in turn causes diarrhea and poor absorption of food. Emil is also a parvo survivor, which could be the cause of the IBD (I didn't know about CS when he had parvo). Flare-ups can be caused by stress or eating something to which he's allergic (he also has multiple food allergies). I give him CS when this happens and it helps eliminate the intestinal bacteria. I use an oral CS and electrolyte solution in a one to ten ratio with one to two ounces of CS. Currently he's recovering from being neutered and I'm putting several ounces of CS in his drinking water every day. He had about three days of post-surgery anesthesia diarrhea, which now has completely cleared up.

Nancy Estes
10211 WCR 52
Midland TX 79707

Colloidal Silver Today

SAFETY

After reviewing the medical literature, the EPA determined that silver is safe to use in moderate amounts. They set an oral Reference Dose (RfD) for silver of 0.005 mg/kg/day. (U.S. EPA, IRIS 1999) This means that someone can ingest that much each day over a seventy-year lifetime with no harmful effects. A man weighing 220 pounds (100 kg) could safely ingest 0.500 mg per day, and a woman weighing 132 pounds (60 kg) could ingest 0.300 mg per day and not go over the RfD.

CS products commercially available today typically contain ten parts per million of silver. This is equivalent to 10 mg of silver per liter (10 mg/l), 2.4 mg per 8 ounce bottle, or 0.050 mg per teaspoon. A 220 pound man could take ten teaspoons of 10 ppm CS per day without exceeding the U.S. EPA's oral Reference Dose.

The critical effect in humans ingesting silver is argyria, a medically benign but permanent bluish-gray discoloration of the skin. Argyria results from the deposition of silver in the dermis and also from silver-induced production of melanin. Although silver has been shown to be uniformly deposited in exposed and unexposed areas, the increased pigmentation becomes more pronounced in areas exposed to sunlight due to photoactivated reduction of the metal. Although the deposition of silver is permanent, it is not associated with any adverse health effects. (U.S. EPA, IRIS 1996)

In the book *Argyria: The Pharmacology of Silver*, the authors reached the conclusion that a total IV dose of 8 gm silver arsphenamine is the limit beyond which argyria may develop. (Hill and Pillsbury, cited by U.S. EPA, IRIS 1996)

32

In my research I have not come across a single report of argyria from the use of 10 ppm CS. There has been no evidence of cancer in humans ever reported from silver exposure despite frequent therapeutic use of the metal over the past one hundred years. (U.S. EPA, IRIS 1996)

Silver can be toxic in large doses, but the concentration of silver for therapeutic doses in CS products used today is quite small. "The estimated fatal dose of silver nitrate is $\geq$ 10 g, but recoveries have been reported following ingestion of larger doses." (Faust 1992)

According to science, silver has no known physiological function in the human body, yet most of us carry around silver in our tissues. The EPA tested twenty-nine samples of human tissue and found silver in 50 percent of them but at lower levels than other trace elements. "Unlike lead or mercury there is no evidence that silver is a cumulative poison." (Petering 1976)

Dosage for CS

There are no published data on dosages for CS because there have been no double blind studies of its effectivness in curing any medical condition. The information on dosages presented below is anecdotal and should not be taken as medical advice.

The Silver Mineral Supplement Ideology

Some people believe that mineral depletion in the world's farming soils has seriously reduced the amount of natural minerals in the average diet necessary to maintain a state of good health. Those who use CS as a mineral supplement generally take about one tablespoon of 5 ppm colloidal silver daily (about 50 micrograms of silver). Taking CS in these small amounts on a daily basis is generally felt to be an illness preventative measure with no associated risks from use. www.silvermedicine.org

Oral Therapeutic Doses

Many people use CS on a need-only basis. Generally, one ounce of 5 to 10 ppm CS is considered one therapeutic dose. How many doses are taken during a twenty-four hour period is quite varied among users. The quantity of doses range from one ounce to sixteen ounces taken daily. Users that practice multiple doses usually take CS three to four times daily, feeling that this produces a sustained and cumulative effect throughout the period of use. However, it may be more beneficial to break down the total daily doses into much more frequent doses, using CS every fifteen minutes to one hour. CS should be held in the mouth at least thirty seconds prior to swallowing. Once symptoms subside, users generally stop taking it. The duration of the treatment for more severe and chronic conditions can be from three weeks to four months and longer. www.silvermedicine.org

Non-Oral Doses

Some users feel that taking CS orally is the least effective method of use. People operating under this ideology use a wide variety of methods to deliver CS into the body, usually in much smaller doses than normally would be taken by ingestion. The operative idea is to deliver the CS into the body in a manner that avoids the digestive system in an attempt to maximize the bio-availability of the silver (for example, via IV or nebulizer). The result is a greater amount of silver working in the body in a less diluted state. www.silvermedicine.org

External CS Use

Colloidal silver often is used externally to address skin conditions and to reduce the spread of bacteria. The general usage philosophy is to apply as needed, since it is widely believed there is is little or no associated risk with external use. Many experienced users believe that the CS must be applied to the area via a dressing or bandage, and therefore keep the bandage hydrated with CS. www.silvermedicine.org

CS AND THE FDA

Sometime in the mid 1980s, a low-voltage direct current (LVDC) method for making CS was developed. When word got out about how easy it was to produce CS, scores of small mom-and-pop businesses began to produce and sell CS and CS generators. There was little quality control and few knew the concentration of silver in the product they were producing. Around this time the Internet began to take off, allowing producers to reach a wider audience and advertise for little cost. Word spread very quickly about this alternative healing product.

The FDA became involved in the CS issue after receiving complaints from a number of sources about the marketing practices of some producers and the quality of the products being sold. They analyzed a number of CS products and found mislabeling and quality issues. Some products did not contain the amount of silver indicated on the label, and some actually had bacteria growing in them. There were assertions made that CS could cure HIV, cancer, and the often repeated claim that it can kill 650 disease bacteria.

The FDA essentially told the industry that their products were misbranded, that they were selling an over-the-counter drug, and that the approval process for introducing a new drug had not been followed. In 1996 the FDA asked for evidence from manufacturers to verify the safety and effectiveness of their CS products. Some producers provided information, but none met the required protocol for such verification and all were rejected.

Much of the information submitted by manufacturers was in the form of testimonials from consumers, but personal experience is not considered by the FDA to be adequate proof of effectiveness or safety. The required protocol to verify safety and effectiveness is very rigorous and can cost a pharmaceutical company hundreds of millions of dollars to conduct. Of course none of the CS manufacturers, who at the time were small business operators, could afford to spend that much money to get their product approved. So the final ruling was issued in August, 1999: drug products containing CS are misbranded and are not generally safe and effective. (See Appendix F for the FDA ruling.)

Some unscrupulous manufacturers are making incredible health claims about CS. While most of these claims have not been verified by scientific research this much is true—**CS kills many common germs very quickly**. Numerous viruses and bacteria are killed within minutes when put in contact with CS. This has been confirmed by a number of independent sources. However, that is in a petri dish. Many in the medical profession are convinced that taking CS is a risk- without-benefit. The concern of many health professionals is that there has been no published scientific research on CS in more than fifty years. Yet thousand of people are using it every day and benefiting from its healing powers. Indeed, some people feel CS has allowed them to lead more normal lives and others feel it has even saved their live's. (See the testimonials on page 22.)

HOMEMADE CS GENERATOR

I have included instructions for a very simple CS generators (with permission from www.silvermedicine.org). It uses four nine-volt batteries. The inventor states that it will produce 3 to 5 ppm CS in less than one hour. The simple electrical parts can be purchased from Radio Shack. Silver wire can be purchased from the sources listed in Appendix D.

SUPPLIES NEEDED

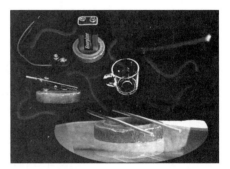

- ✔ 4 nine-volt alkaline batteries. These are needed to achieve the desired thirty volts of electricity. (Although four batteries in series total thiry-six volts, the drain on the batteries quickly brings the total voltage down to thirty.)

- ✔ 2 nine-volt battery connectors

- ✔ 2 metal alligator clips

- ✔ 1 glass beaker or container that comfortably holds eight ounces of fluid

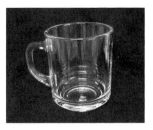

- ✔ 2 fine silver rods (9 cm rods shown, minimum 14 gauge) or two strips of 18 gauge fine silver wire. Any silver used must be at least 99.9 percent pure.

ADDITIONAL SUPPLIES NEEDED

- ✔ 1 gallon of distilled water (Walgreens and Arrowhead are two recommended brands)

- ✔ 1 roll of pure white paper towels

- ✔ 1 pure nylon scrub pad (the green Scotch Brite pads)

- ✔ 1 glass container in which to store the colloidal silver (UV protected glass is recommended)

PREPARING THE BATTERY SETUP

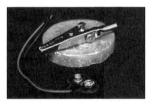

You will need two nine-volt battery connectors. Attach the alligator clips to the nine-volt battery connector leads according to the following instructions.

Attach one alligator clip to the red (positive) wire of the battery connector, and one alligator clip to the black (negative) wire of the other battery connector. Strip off about one-quarter inch of insulation from the end of the wire and securely attach the lead to the alligator clip under the screw. Clip off the unused wire on each connector. You should now have two battery connectors with an alligator clip attached to each one. (See photograph.)

Attach the battery pairs as shown in the photograph: Take two nine-volt batteries and snap the positive pole of one to the negative pole of the other. There is only one way that this attachment will work. Repeat the process for the second set of batteries. The end result will be two sets of two batteries attached to each other.

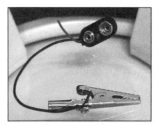

Attach the two battery sets together: (Do not perform this step until you are actually prepared to make your colloidal silver. Once the four batteries are attached, a circuit will be completed). Take the two battery sets and snap them together. The end result will be four batteries attached together. Note: To avoid a potential hazard created by alkaline batteries wired in series, any concerned user may wire a twenty-four-volt light bulb in series. However, we have never heard of a problem with the batteries exploding.

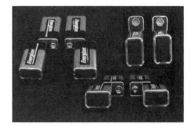

COMPLETING THE HOOKUP

The final step is to attach the battery leads. Attach the positive (red) battery connector to the exposed positive pole on the batteries. Attach the nega-tive (black) battery connector to the exposed negative pole

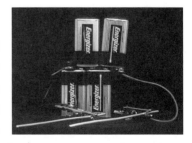

of the batteries. To test the connection, tap the two alligator clips together to see if a small spark is generated. There is only one way to attach the connectors to the batteries, so do not be concerned about not attaching them properly.

NOW THE BASIC GENERATOR ASSEMBLY SHOULD BE COMPLETE. THE REMAINING STEPS WILL PREPARE THE GLASS AND SILVER RODS FOR USE.

Wash your hands thoroughly.

Use the nylon scrub pad and dry scrub the inside of your glass container.

Rinse the container thoroughly. Use a clean paper towel to dry the container. Rinse a second time with a small amount of distilled water.

Always scrub the silver wire or rods with a nylon scrub pad before use. To avoid wasting silver, use light pressure and agitate quickly. The smoothness of the electrodes will help to ensure a uniform draw of ions from the silver rod.

Wipe off the rods with a clean paper towel dampened with a small amount of distilled water.

Add approximately eight ounces of distilled water to the glass container.

Assemble the colloidal silver generator as previously described by attaching the two battery sets together. (Never leave the generator assembled when it is not in use).

THE PREPARATION OF THE SILVER RODS AND GLASS IS NOW COMPLETE. THE NEXT STEP IS THE BREW PROCESS.

Position the rods above the container. Any clean, non-conductive material may be used. For example you can use two chopsticks clamped together at the ends with rubber bands. (See the following photographs.)

Attach the alligator clips to the silver rods. Position the battery setup so that both of the attached rods may be easily

inserted in the water. For optimum performance, the spacing between the rods should be one and one-half to two inches. The rods should be positioned as close to the center of the container as possible to prevent increased conductivity along the rim of the container.

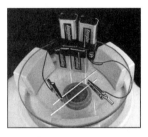

Position the rods parallel to each other. This encourages uniform conductivity between both rods, and therefore a uniform draw of silver. The positive and negative leads/rods should never touch each other.

Once the alligator clips are connected to the silver rods, record the time. As the batch pro-

gresses through the first ten to fifteen minutes, very little change should be apparent. As the fifteen-minute mark approaches, pay particular attention to the reaction.

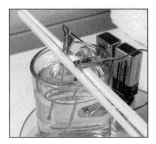

After about fifteen to thirty minutes, you should notice a thin yellow cloud or a yellow wisp drifting between the electrodes. This indicates that the concentration of silver ions between both rods is reaching a point of ideal saturation. Record the time.

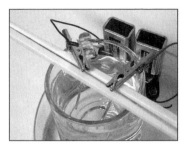

Allow the reaction to continue for five minutes. Then, very carefully, remove the negative rod from the water. Wait about two minutes. Gently remove the positive rod from the water. Disconnect the alligator clips from the silver rods and disassemble the batteries.

Increasing the brew time will increase the concentration of the end colloidal silver. However, be aware that you risk degrading the product. You can use a Hanna PWT meter to measure the ionic content of silver (as well as the initial quality of the distilled water). You also can use the salt test to determine ionic content. (See page 53.) A laser pen in a dark room can be used to gauge the amount of particulate silver in the end product. (This is the Tyndall effect. See page 17.)

You may notice the remaining yellow wisps slowly dissipating. As time progresses, the colloidal silver will retain its clear "water" color. No visible particles should be present. Increasing the production time will eventually result in colloidal silver with a yellow hue.

With this method, every single batch of CS will have a different ppm reading, but if the above instructions are followed, the end product's silver concentration will be three to five parts per million. The particle size will be between .001 and .04 microns in diameter.

Note: Nylon is used to clean the silver rods and glass because it is a non-reactive substance and any accidental contamination will not interfere with the reaction. It is also a nontoxic substance.

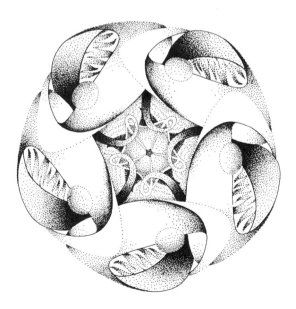

MASTERING COLLOIDAL SILVER PRODUCTION

The ability to produce a good quality CS is dependent on three factors: purity, current control, and timing.

Purity: The quality of any colloidal silver is foremost determined by the purity of the silver used, the purity of the initial water supply, and the cleanliness of both the silver rods and the glass container used for production. Even variables such as air quality and light concentration can influence colloidal silver production.

Current Control: The entire colloidal silver generation process is geared toward strict regulation of the flow of silver (both ions and particles) into the distilled water base. The more one can successfully control this, the higher the quality will be. Variable conditions include everything covered in the purity principle plus the following: the voltage applied, the amount of current, the size and the shape of the silver electrodes, the amount of water used, the water temperature, the size and shape of the container, the shape of the silver electrodes, the spacing between the silver rods, the motion (if any) of the water in the container, and even the Earth's electromagnetic field.

Timing: Understanding and properly measuring the duration of each batch of colloidal silver is of paramount importance to both the particle size of the silver ions and the concentration of the batch itself. Thus it is critical to the end quality of the product. Timing influences particle sizing and particle dispersion (known as 'hydration of the silver').

Each of these three principles relies upon the other. Mastery of these simple principles equates to mastery of colloidal silver production. Every advanced colloidal silver generator is advanced due to the fact that it addresses these principles successfully. www.silvermedicine.org

I would recommend that you have your home-brewed CS tested before using it. The cost is about $25.00. (See Appendix D for a list of companies.)

CONCLUSION

By now you should have a clear understanding of CS and its uses. The anecdotal evidence for CS's effectiveness is amazing. Thousands of people are using it to treat a variety of ailments from minor cuts to serious diseases. Many people are making CS at home and feel empowered by their freedom from the medical establishment. Meanwhile, the government and drug companies continue to express no interest in CS.

Currently, there are no industry standards for the manufacture of CS and no quality control for what is being sold. A wise consumer will shop carefully and choose CS from manufacturers that test their product regularly. Look for a published analysis of parts per million (ppm) silver content that includes a measure of both silver particles and silver ions.

As discussed earlier, some researchers insist that the most effective CS has the highest percentage of the smallest possible silver particles, and a low percentage of dissolved silver ions. Others say that it's the silver ions that do the healing and that ionic silver is the most effective.

Most CS today is produced by the low voltage, direct current (LVDC) method that generally contains 10 percent colloidal silver particles and 90 percent dissolved silver ions. Many people are using this ionic- colloidal silver successfully. You will have to do your own research to determine where you stand on the issue of particles vs. ions.

With all the use of CS these days I have yet to come across a report of a serious reaction from someone using 10 ppm colloidal silver. (There is sometimes a temporary flu-like reaction called a "Jarisch-Herxheimer effect." As the disease microorganisms die off, they release toxins that need to be eliminated from the body.) I have not come across a report of anyone getting argyria from using 10 ppm CS. From the anecdotal evidence it seems that people are being cured by CS. There are thousands of people who are being helped by it and who believe in its healing powers.

Silver in the form of CS is assured a place in history as a powerful germ killer. Today CS is readily available, and with its low-tech production process and broad spectrum germicidal properties, it could be an important healing tool worldwide, especially in the third world. There is clear historic evidence that CS is effective in killing disease microbes. There is compelling modern evidence that CS is an effective germ killer.

It is time for government funded research on colloidal silver—carefully monitored studies to determine its safety and effectiveness in curing disease.

If you want to learn more about CS from people who are using it and reasearching it, join the silver-list chat group listed in Appendix E.

APPENDIX A. WHAT IS A COLLOIDAL SUBSTANCE?

I have included the following extended excerpts from Professor James B. Calvert's writing on colloids posted on his Web site. Dr. Calvert is Associate Professor Emeritus of Engineering, University of Denver, and a Registered Professional Engineer in the state of Colorado.

"Colloids are sometimes referred to as a 'fourth state of matter.' It is easy to recognize the three conventional states of matter in ice, water and steam. The terms *solid, liquid* and *gas* can be attached to certain suites of properties, and make useful distinctions. Many substances can be classified by these properties, but the terms do not separate matter into three mutually exclusive catagories and may not be descriptive enough. Where is tar, for example, or jelly? Colloids provide many examples of substances for which the simple classification into three states is wholly inadequate.

"The most significant property of colloids is their large surface area. To some degree, they are all surface and their properties are those of their surfaces. I shall use the word 'colloid' to refer to both a substance of colloidal dimensions as well as a colloidal system.

"Consider a substance in the form of a cube that is one cubic centimeter in size. In this form, it has an area of 0.0006 m². We could say that it is almost all volume. Most of its molecules safely reside behind its surface, secure from disturbance or attack. Let us now divide it into thin laminae, 10 nm thick, a colloidal distance. The cube becomes one million laminae, with a total surface area of 200 m². Every molecule is now only a short distance from the harsh elements, and the material is all surface. We have turned the mass cube into a laminated colloid by this delicate slicing alone.

"Continuing, we now slice each of the million laminae into one million fibers, and the surface area doubles. Finally, each fiber is chopped into one million bits, giving a corpuscular colloid. This increases the surface area by 50 percent, to 600 m². From the original mass to the corpuscle, the surface area has been increased by a factor of one million, which is typical of a colloid.

"The large area emphasizes surface effects relative to volume effects, giving colloids different properties than those of bulk matter. It is better to define a colloid as a system in which the surface area is large and in which surface effects are predominant, rather than simply in terms of particle size. Indeed, in foams there are no colloidal particles at all—it is the thinness of the films that creates the colloidal behavior. A colloid is a material system that is mainly surface.

"The next important characteristic is that a colloid is, at the minimum, a two-phase system. A phase is a homogeneous component of a system. A colloidal system consists of an internal phase, which is the material of colloidal dimensions, and an external phase, which is the material in which the colloid is dispersed. These designations are analogous to the terms *solute* and *solvent* used for simple solutions (which form a single phase). As the particles of a corpuscular colloid become smaller and smaller, they imperceptibly trancend from a two-phase colloid to a single-phase solution, with no definite boundary.

"The colloidal system that is most similar to a simple solution is a dispersion of corpuscles, or particles, in a liquid. This is called a *sol*, and the liquid is the external phase. This is the classical colloid as described by Graham [and our colloidal silver]. If the external phase is a solid instead of a liquid, the system is called a *solid sol*. The only difference is the mobility of the molecules. In a solid sol, they can move only by diffusion. If the external phase is a gas, usually air, instead of a liquid, we have an aerosol. There is no definite boundary between a sol and a solution, but still they are significantly different. There also is no definite boundary between a sol and a coarse suspension. A coarse suspension will settle out rapidly, while a sol may be permanent.

"The particles that appear in a sol may or may not be wetted by the liquid. Wetting is a typical surface effect, and it is of paramount importance in a colloid system. With wetting, the liquid is adsorbed on the surface of the particle. The terms *adsorb* and *absorb* may sound alike, but their meanings are quite different. A substance that is absorbed is taken into the volume of the absorbing substance, as is water when mixed with sand. If a substance is adsorbed, it attaches itself only to the surface. Because colloids are all surface, adsorption is what is important when working with them. If the particle adsorbs the external phase, it is called *lyophilic*, or *hydrophilic*, if the external phase is water. The Greek verb *luo* means to dissolve or destroy, and *philic* is derived from *philos* which means love. A lyophilic colloid 'loves the external phase.' On the other hand, if the particle does not adsorb the external phase, it is said to be *lyophobic*, or 'fears the external phase.'

"Sols that contain inorganic particles, such as metals, are mostly lyophobic, as are most aerosols and solid sols. Lyophobic hydrosols are a very common kind of colloid and deserve a detailed description. For example, consider the hydrosol of gold with particles about 4 nm in size. This was one of the first sols to be studied extensively, and it has interesting properties. With about 0.1 percent gold, the sol is a rich ruby red. The similar solid sol in glass makes ruby glass. The gold particles absorb strongly in the green and blue, so the transmitted light is red. If the gold particles clump together, which they may do over time, the color of the solution changes. When the particles are about 40 nm in diameter, the solution is blue, with considerable scattered light. If the particles agglomerate further, the color disappears and gold flakes settle out.

"Bacteria can be suspended in water to form a sol, which has all the classic properties. The Brownian motion, the Tyndall effect (turbidity), and even electrophoresis are seen. The bacteria act as a hydrophobic sol, peptized by their electrostatic charge. The properties of a sol are largely independent of the nature of the internal phase.

Colloidal Silver Today

"There are two interesting questions that need to be addressed about the stability of the sol. First, what keeps the gold suspended in the red solution so the tiny particles do not settle out? The gold particles fall under gravity through the water. At the same time, the particles are subject to the bombardment of the molecules of the liquid, which produces the Brownian movement. For a sufficiently small particle, the upward diffusion produced by the Brownian movement overcomes the gravitational fall, and an equilibrium is reached, much like the equilibrium of gases in the atmosphere. There is a critical size for a particle, below which it will not settle out.

"Second, how are the particles kept from agglomerating? Generally, if two colloidal particles collide, they will stick together and make a bigger particle, because this is usually favored by energy. Eventually, the particles get larger than the critical size necessary to be suspended by the Brownian movement and they settle out. There must be some good reason if this is not to happen. In most lyophobic colloids [such as colloidal silver water], the particles are electrically charged with the same sign. This keeps them apart because they repel each other. The particles are charged mainly because they adsorb certain ions in the environment. In water, these may be OH- ions, which generally are present and give the particles a negative charge. The H+ ions are hydrated, so they are not as easy to adsorb, but apparently some particles like them and become positively charged. If you try to make a hydrosol with particles of opposite charges, they neutralize each other and the sol collapses. Since lyophobic sols are stabilized by an electric charge, adding electrolytes generally destroys the sol. When rivers reach the sea with their loads of colloidal sediment, the ions in sea water coagulate the sol and the load is deposited in the delta.

"How the charges are distributed is an interesting subject. The sol appears electrically neutral on the large scale. The particle with its adsorbed charges is called a granule. The charges are in a thin layer on the surface. They attract an atmosphere of opposite charges from the external phase, just as an electron in a plasma surrounds itself with a shielding positive charge by attracting positive ions and repelling electrons. The whole neutral structure—granule plus mobile external charge—is called a micelle. This, then, is what moves around—the charged particle and its cloud of opposite charge. When we apply an electric field to the sol, the cloud of charge is moved in one direction and the granule moves in the other. There is a local viscous flow about the granule, and the micelle moves toward the anode, if the granule is positive, or toward the cathode, if it is negative. This movement is called electrophoresis and can be practically useful. Because of the shielding, the particles of a sol do not repel each other until they come quite close and their micelles overlap.

"In order to create a lyophobic sol, a mass must be reduced to colloidal size, called *dispersion*, or the colloidal particles must be built from molecules, called *condensation*. In either case, a third substance, a peptizing agent, may need to be added to stabilize the sol. Dispersion can be done mechanically in a colloid mill that grinds the substance into small, equal particles. Another method is with an electric arc. In this case, metal electrodes are used at a current of 5 to 10A and voltage of 30 to 40V. Bredig made particles of about 40 nm by this method, and it was improved by Svedburg to obtain sols of many metals down to 5 nm particle size. Ultrasonics also can be used to disperse sols.

"One common effect of colloids is turbidity, an effect like that of stirring up mud in water. Slight turbidity may not be noticed until a beam of light passes through the colloid. Colloidal systems need not be turbid: a gel may be quite transparent when the particles are small. Solutions, as with homogeneous phases, are not turbid. The turbidity causes scattering so that the path of the light beam can be clearly seen. This is called the Tyndall effect, and the observed scattered light is called the Tyndall cone. All the Tyndall cones that you see are evidence of lyophobic sols." (Hartman cited by Calvet 2003)

51

APPENDIX B.

The author of this paper, Frank Key, has spent thousands of hours performing research in the science of colloids and the production of metal colloids in particular. He has built a laboratory facility for colloidal research which is state of the art for the field. He also manufactures and sells CS.

COLLOIDAL SILVER BY FRANK KEY

Ions, Atoms and Charged Particles

"Many non-scientific writers confuse *ions* and *charged particles* and use the terms interchangeably when describing colloidal silver. Others refer to colloidal particles as though they are single atoms of silver. Much has been written about silver particles having a positive charge, which is false. It is no wonder then that lay people trying to learn about colloidal silver become confused and have a hard time grasping the science involved with the subject matter when so much of what they read is scientifically flawed. Since the real science involved in understanding colloidal suspensions requires an understanding of the underlying principles, it is important to have a clear understanding of the differences between atoms, ions and charged particles.

Silver Ions

"A silver ion is a single atom of silver that is missing one electron from its outer orbit. The diameter of a silver ion is 0.230 nm, which is slightly smaller than an atom owing to one less electron. The missing electron causes the ion to be positively charged and also changes the physical properties in some very dramatic ways. Metallic silver is not soluble in water, but ionic silver has a finite measurable solubility. Typically, silver is dissolved in an acid such as nitric acid to form silver nitrate. When silver is dissolved, it is no longer metallic silver. It is not visible even under the most powerful microscope and it does not reflect light. Even a solution saturated with Ag+ ions has no Tyndall effect, but colloidal Ag does, even in concentrations as little as 0.1 ppm. The solubility product constant, Ksp for AgOH is 1.52×10^{-8}, which means that, in a neutral solution, one could have 9.2×10^{22} Ag ions per liter without getting precipitation.

"In summary, a silver ion is positively charged because it lacks an electron. An electron has a negative charge. Take away an electron and the ion so formed assumes a positive charge. The charge attributed to ions is ionic charge and it is due to the gain or loss of electrons. This is not the same as a particle that may have a charge. Particle charge is due to the adsorption of charged species. In fact the silver particles found in colloidal silver are negatively charged, not positive like the ions.

Simple Demonstration of Ionic Silver

"To demonstrate ionic silver content, all that is needed is a chloride ion source to be added to a small amount of colloidal silver. Normal table salt is sodium chloride (NaCl). When table salt is dissolved in water it decomposes into sodium ions and chloride ions. To demonstrate place a small amount (one to two ounces) of colloidal silver in a clear glass. Add a few grains of table salt. Observe that as the salt dissolves a white cloud of silver chloride forms in the solution. Eventually the entire solution will turn cloudy. If more salt is added, the white silver chloride will become denser until all the silver ions have combined with the available chlorine ions. If no silver ions are present, no white cloud will form.

How CS is Produced Today

"Colloidal silver generally is produced by electrolysis when an electric current is passed through a series circuit consisting of a silver electrode and de-ionized (DI) water. The current can be either alternating current (AC) or direct current (DC). The current flow causes Ag0 (metal) and Ag+ (ions) to migrate from the electrode into the

DI water. AC processes tend to be more efficient than DC in limiting the ionic concentration. It generally is assumed that water ionizes to H+ and OH-, and that the H+, in the form of the hydronium ion, H_3O+, migrates to the cathode, where it is reduced to hydrogen gas, H_2, which is liberated. The electrons taken from the cathode are replaced at the anode when Ag metal goes into solution as Ag+.

"Therefore, colloidal silver consists of silver in two distinctly different forms, metallic silver particles and ions. The total amount of silver that is reported as the silver concentration (in parts per million) is the sum total of the silver contained in the particles and the silver contained in the silver ions. Accurate measurement of the total silver content requires the measurement by either atomic absorption or atomic emission of the silver atoms. An Atomic Absorption Spectrophotometer (AAS) is typically used for accurate results. To measure the concentration of silver ions by atomic absorption requires that the particles first be removed by centrifugation leaving only the ions.

The Physics Involved in CS Production

"How does electrolysis produce silver particles? This discussion of electrolysis assumes two silver electrodes are placed in deionized water a small distance apart. The electrodes are connected to a low voltage DC power source (9 to 30 VDC). The electrode connected to the positive (+) terminal is referred to as the anode, the electrode connected to the negative (-) terminal is referred to as the cathode.

"When electric current passes through silver, some silver atoms at the interface with the water will lose an electron changing the atom into an ion. Whereas metallic silver is not water soluble, silver ions are water soluble, so the silver ions simply dissolve in the water producing an ionic silver solution. This is the electrolysis process. With the electrolysis process, some of the ions in close proximity to the anode will take on an electron from the current passing through and be changed from an ion back into an atom. These atoms are attracted by other similar atoms by Van der Waal's force of attraction and thus form small metallic particles. This is how both ions and particles are produced by the electrolysis process.

"Typically 90 percent of the silver leaving the anode stays in the ionic form while about 10 percent forms into particles. Furthermore, a silver ion is not a group of atoms; rather, it is a single silver atom that is missing a single electron. Silver ions remain dispersed in the solution from other silver ions due to their positive 'ionic charge' which causes mutual repulsion. The silver particles do not have a positive charge. Their charge is negative and is not due to 'ionic charge' as are the ions. Instead they have a zeta potential which causes the particle to act as though it had a negative charge.

"Two silver ions will not get close together until an electron is added to each ion to convert it back to an atom. Only atoms can join together to form particles. Atoms do not have a charge and thus no mutual repulsion is created. Ions in close proximity will have a repulsive force of well over one hundred thousand G-forces causing them to mutually repel each other. There is no force strong enough to overcome this force. Brownian motion is not sufficient." (Key 2000)

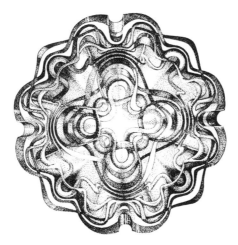

APPENDIX C. SILVER AND TISSUE REGENERATION

Here is a patented system using silver to produce tissue regeneration.

United States Patent 5,814,094 Becker, et al. September 29, 1998 Iontopheretic system for stimulation of tissue healing and regeneration

"Abstract: An iontophoretic system for promoting tissue healing processes and inducing regeneration. The system includes a device and a method, a composition, and methods for making the composition in vitro and in vivo. The system is implemented by placing a flexible, silver-containing anode in contact with the wound, placing a cathode on intact skin near the anode, and applying a wound-specific DC voltage between the anode and the cathode. Electrically-generated silver ions from the anode penetrate into the adjacent tissues and undergo a sequence of reactions leading to formation of a silver-collagen complex. This complex acts as a biological inducer to cause the formation in vivo of an adequate blastema to support regeneration."

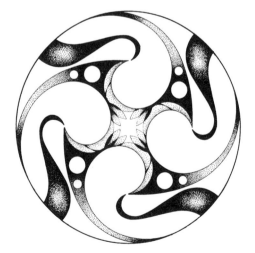

APPENDIX D. COLLOIDAL SILVER TESTING

You can get your colloidal silver tested by contacting the following companies:

Natural-Immunogenics Inc.
7440 SW 50th Terrace Unit 107
Miami, FL 33155
305-669-0233
sales@natural-immunogenics.com

Colloidal Science Laboratory, Inc.
213 Irick Rd.
Westampton, NJ 08060
866-233-4633
4info@purestcolloids.com

PII
3516 Delilah Dr.
Cape Coral, FL 33993
239-283-8640
www.health2us.com

You also can get a fairly accurate test with the use of a PWT meter available from select companies that sell CS.

Silver wire can be purchased from the following companies:

Advent Research Materials http://www.advent-rm.com

www.ccsilver.com

Hauser & Miller Co.
10950 Lin Valle Dr.
St. Louis, MO 63123
800-462-7447

APPENDIX E.
SOURCES FOR CS, CS GENERATORS,
AND INFORMATION

www.americanbiotechlabs.com

www.colloidalsilvergens.com

www.colloidal-silver.com

www.health2us.com

www.natural-immunogenics.com

www.purestcolloids.com.

www.silver-colloids.com

www.silvergen.com

www.silverlist.org (a moderated chat group for people who make or use CS)

www.silvermedicine.org

www.silverpuppy.com

www.utopiasilver.com

To order a copy of Albert Searle's book *The Use of Colloids in Health and Disease,* contact:

Borderland Science Research Foundation
P.O. Box 6250
Eureka, CA 95502
707-445-2247

APPENDIX F. THE FDA's FINAL RULING ON CS

FDA ISSUES FINAL RULE ON OTC DRUG PRODUCTS CONTAINING COLLOIDAL SILVER

The FDA has issued a Final Rule declaring that all over-the-counter (OTC) drug products containing colloidal silver or silver salts are not recognized as safe and effective and are misbranded.

Colloidal silver is a suspension of silver particles in a colloidal (gelatinous) base. In recent years, colloidal silver preparations of unknown formulation have been appearing in stores. These products are labeled to treat adults and children for diseases including HIV, AIDS, cancer, tuberculosis, malaria, lupus, syphilis, scarlet fever, shingles, herpes, pneumonia, typhoid, tetanus and many others.

According to the Final Rule, a colloidal silver product for any drug use will first have to be approved by FDA under the new drug application procedures. The Final Rule classifies colloidal silver products as misbranded because adequate directions cannot be written so that the general public can use these drugs safely for their intended purposes. They are also misbranded when their labeling falsely suggests that there is substantial scientific evidence to establish that the drugs are safe and effective for their intended uses.

The indiscriminate use of colloidal silver solutions has resulted in cases of argyria, a permanent blue-gray discoloration of the skin and deep tissues.

Colloidal silver ingredients and silver salts include silver proteins, mild silver protein, strong silver protein, silver chloride, and silver iodide. The dosage form of these colloidal silver products is usually oral, but product labeling also contains directions for topical and, occasionally, intravenous use.

In reaching its decision, FDA considered all of the information described in the proposed rule (October 15, 1996) and submitted by the public in response to that proposal, the Final Rule becomes effective on September 16, 1999, 30 days after publication.

REFERENCES

(ATSDR), "Toxicological profile for silver," Agency for Toxic Substances and Disease Registry, Atlanta, 1990, cited by Faust.

(ATSDR), "Silver Fact Sheet," CAS#7440-22-4, Agency for Toxic Substances and Disease Registry, Atlanta, 1999.

(APUA), Alliance For The Prudent Use Of Antibiotics, APUA Newsletter 17(3): 1-3, 1999.

Bakteriol, Zentralbl, "Antimicrobial activity and biocompatibility of polyurethane and silicone catheters containing low concentrations of silver: a new perspective in prevention of polymer-associated foreign-body-infections," 1995.

Becker, United States Patent, 5,814,094 Becker, et al., September 29, "Iontopheretic system for stimulation of tissue healing and regeneration," 1998.

Calvert, James B., "Colloids," 2003. on the Internet at: www.du.edu/~jcalvert/phys/colloid.htm

Chambers, Krieger J, et al., "Silver ion inhibition of serine proteases: Crystallographic study of silver- trypsin," *Biochem.and Biophys. Res. Comm.*, 59, 70-74, 1974, cited by WHO.

Cooper, C. F. and W. C. Jolly, "Ecological effects of silver iodide and other weather modification agents; A review," *Water Resources Research*, 6, 88-98, 1970, cited by WHO.

Crookes, Henry, "On Metallic Colloids and Their Bactericidal Properties: The History of Collosols." *Scientific American*, July 1914.

Faust, Rosmarie A., "Toxicity Summary for Silver" Chemical Hazard Evaluation and Communication Group, Biomedical and Environmental Information Analysis Section, Health and Safety Research Division, Oak Ridge National Laboratory, Oak Ridge, 1992.

Fung, Man C., et al., "Silver Products for Medical Uses," 1996.

------, et al., "Silver indications: risk-benefit assessment," *Journal of Toxicology: Clinical Toxicology*; 34(1):119-26, 1995.

Gaul, L.E., and A.H, Staud, "Clinical spectroscopy: Seventy cases of generalized argyria following organic and colloidal silver medication," *J. Am. Med. Assoc.* 104: 1387-1390, 1935, cited by Faust.

Gibbs, Ronald J., *Silver Colloids, Do They Work?*, unpublished book, 1990.

Hamilton, E.I., and M.J. Minski, "Abundance of the chemical elements in man's diet and possible relations with environmental factors," *Sci. Total Environ.*, 1: 375-394, 1972, cited by WHO.

Hartman, R. J., *Colloid Chemistry*, Pitman and Sons, London, 1949, cited by James B. Calvert, www.du.edu/~jcalvert/index.htm

Hill, John W., *Colloidal Silver, A Literature Review: Medical Uses, Toxicology, and Manufacture, Edition 2*, unpublished paper, 2000.

Hill, W.R., and D.M. Pillsbury, *Argyria: The Pharmacology of Silver*, Williams and Wilkins Company, Baltimore, 1939.

Kehoe, R. D., et al., "A spectrochemical study of the normal ranges of concentrations of certain trace metals in biological materials," *J. Nutrit.*, *19*, 579-592, 1940, cited by WHO.

Key, Francis S. and George Maass, *Silver Colloids*, unpublished paper, www.silver-colloids.com, 2000.

Klaus, T., et al., "Silver-based crystalline nanoparticles, microbially fabricated," PNAS 96, 13611-13614, *Lancet*, 235-240, 1999.

NIAID, "Antimicrobial Resistance Fact Sheet," National Inst. of Allergies & Infectious Diseases, National Inst. of Health, Bethesda.

Nordberg, G. F. and L. Gerhardsson, "Silver," *Handbook on Toxicity of Inorganic Compounds*, H.G. Seiler and H. Sigel, eds. Marcel Dekker, Inc., New York, 1988, pp. 619-623, cited by Faust.

Petering, H. G., "Pharmacology and toxicology of heavy metals: silver," *Pharmac. Ther. A.*, *1*, 127-130, 1976, cited by WHO.

Colloidal Silver Today

Schramm, Laurier L., *The Dictionary of Colloidal & Interface Science*, Wiley-Interscience, New York, 2001.

Searle, Albert, *The Use of Colloids in Health and Disease*, Contable & Company LTD, London, 1919.

The Silver Institute, 1112 16th St., N.W. , Suite 240, Washington, DC, 20039, 202-835-0185, fax: 202-835-0155.

Silver, S., et al., "Silver cations as an antimicrobial agent: clinical uses and bacterial resistance," 1999, cited by Alliance For The Prudent Use Of Antibiotics, APUA Newsletter 17(3): 1-3, 1999.

Sioshansi, P., Spire Corporation, Bedford, Mass. 01730-2396, PMID: 8024473 (PubMed—indexed for MEDLINE).

Stokinger, H.E. "Silver," *Patty's Industrial Hygiene and Toxicology, vol. 2A*, G.D. Clayton and E. Clayton, eds., John Wiley & Sons, New York, pp. 1881-1894, 1981, cited by Faust.

Tripton, I. H. and Cook, M. J., "Trace elements in human tissue, Part II. Adult subjects from the United States," *Health Phys.*, 9, 103-145, 1963, cited by WHO.

U. S. FDA, (1996) "Over-the-counter drug products containing colloidal silver ingredients or silver salts," Federal Register, October 15, 61(200): 53685-53688; US Food and Drug Administration, FDA Health Fraud Bulletin #19, Colloidal Silver, October 7, 1994.

U. S. EPA, "Drinking Water Criteria Document for Silver" (Final Draft), 1985. Environmental Criteria and Assessment Office, Cincinnati, ECAO-CIN-026, PB86-118288, cited by Faust.

U.S. EPA IRIS, Integrated Risk Information System, "Silver;" (CASRN 7440-22-4), 1996

World Health Organization (WHO), "Summary of Toxicological Data of Certain Food Additives," on the Internat at: www.inchem.org/documents/jecfa/jecmono/v12je19.htm

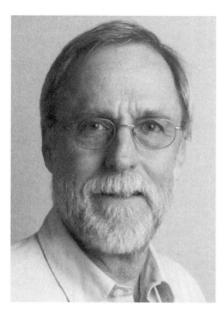

Warren Jefferson has been interested in alternative health practices since first becoming a vegetarian in 1967. He works as an art director, photographer, and research writer for the Book Publishing Company, which specializes in books on vegetarian cookbooks, alternative health, and Native American culture. He has edited and worked on numerous publications on a variety of subjects.

Warren's first book, *The World of Chief Seattle,* is an historical account of Chief Seattle's people the Suquamish from pre-contact time to the present. It includes the Suquamish authorized version of Chief Seattle's speech. The book was written in cooperation with the Suquamish, and they receive a portion of the royalties.

His third book, *The Neti Pot for Better Health,* gives all the information one needs to use this traditional health care tool to relieve allergies and sinus problems.

Warren and his wife Barbara are founding members of the Farm Community in Tennessee, which is dedicated to ecology, vegetarianism, natural childbirth, and nonviolence. They have four children who were all raised vegetarian.

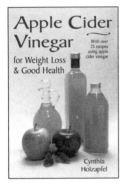
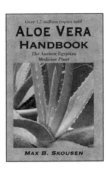
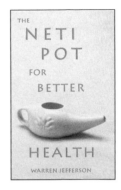
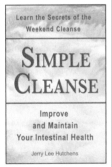
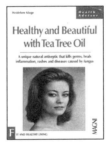
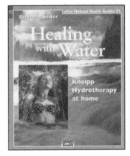